Active at Any Size

WOULD you like to be more physically active, but are not sure if you can do it?

Good news—if you are a very large person, **you _can_ be physically active**—and you can have fun and feel good doing it.

THERE may be special challenges for very large people who are physically active. You may not be able to bend or move in the same way that other people can. It may be hard to find clothes and equipment for exercising. You may feel self-conscious being physically active around other people.

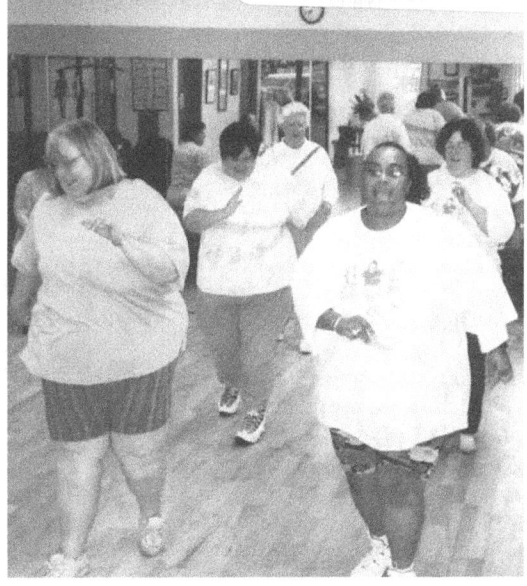

Facing these challenges is hard—but it can be done! The information in this booklet may help you start being more active and healthier—**no matter what your size!**

Why should I be active?

BEING physically active may help you **live longer** and protect you from:

- type 2 diabetes
- heart disease
- stroke
- high blood pressure

If you have any of these health problems, being physically active may help improve your symptoms.

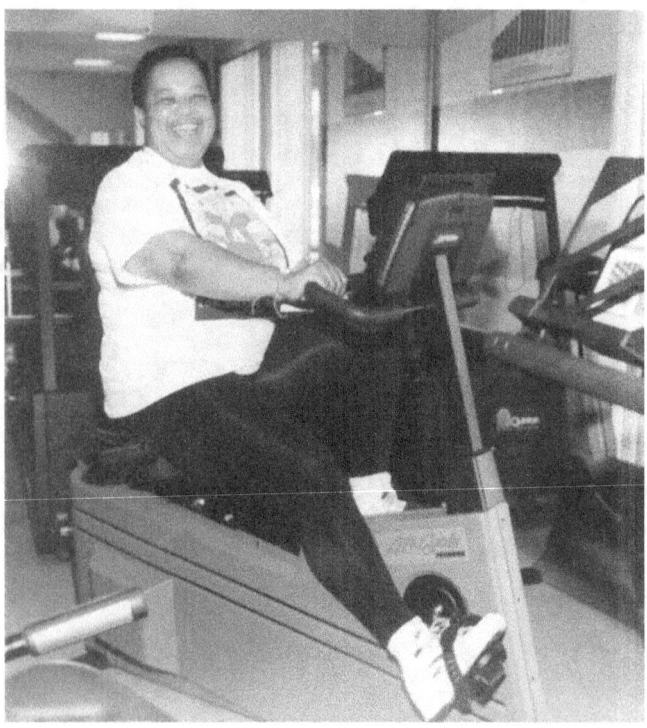

Being physically active can be a lot of fun!

REGULAR physical activity helps you **feel better** because it:

- Lowers your stress and boosts your mood.
- Increases your strength, movement, balance, and flexibility.
- Helps control blood pressure and blood sugar.
- Helps build healthy bones, muscles, and joints.
- Helps your heart and lungs work better.
- Improves your self-esteem.
- Boosts energy during the day and may aid in sleep at night.

How do I get started?

TO start being more active, try these tips:

- **Think about your barriers to being active.** Then try to come up with creative ways to solve them. The following examples may help you overcome barriers.

> Barrier: **I don't have enough time!**
>
> Solution: Be active for a few minutes at a time throughout the day. Sit less. Try to walk more while doing your errands, or schedule lunchtime workouts to boost your overall activity. Plan ahead and be creative!

Barrier: **I feel self-conscious when I'm active.**

Solution: Be active at home while doing household chores, and find ways to move more during your day-to-day activities. Try walking with a group of friends with whom you feel comfortable.

Barrier: **I'm worried about my health or injury.**

Solution: You might feel better if you talk to a health care professional first. Find a fitness provider to guide you, or sign up for a class so you feel safe. Remember that activity does not have to be difficult! Gentle activity is good too.

Barrier: **I just don't like exercise.**

Solution: Good news—you do not have to run or do push-ups to get the benefits of being physically active. Try dancing to the radio, walking outdoors, or being active with friends to spice things up.

Barrier: **I can't stay motivated!**

Solution: Try to add variety to your activities and ask your friends to help you stay focused on being active. Consider an activity video for extra encouragement. Also, set realistic goals, track your progress, and be sure to celebrate your achievements!

- **Start slowly.** Your body needs time to get used to your new activity.

- **Warm up.** Warm-ups get your body ready for action. Shrug your shoulders, tap your toes, swing your arms, or march in place. Walk more slowly for the first few minutes.

- **Cool down.** Slow down little by little. If you have been walking fast, walk slowly for a few minutes to cool down. Cooling down may protect your heart, relax your muscles, and keep you from getting hurt.

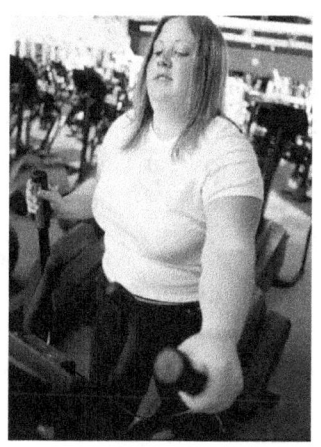

Appreciate yourself!

If you cannot do an activity, do not be hard on yourself. Feel good about what you **can** do. Be proud of pushing yourself up out of a chair or walking a short distance.

Pat yourself on the back for **trying** even if you cannot do it the first time. It may be easier the next time!

How do I continue to be active?

To maintain your active lifestyle, try these suggestions:

◆ **Pledge to be active.** Making a commitment to yourself to be active may help you stay motivated, stay on track, and reach your goals. Consider using the activity pledge at the end of this booklet to help you start and continue to be active.

◆ **Set goals.** Set short-term and long-term goals. A short-term goal may be to walk 5 to 10 minutes, 5 days a week. It may not seem like a lot, but any activity is better than none. A long-term goal may be to do at least 30 minutes of physical activity at a moderate-intensity level (one that makes you breathe harder but does not overwork or overheat you) on most days of the week. You can break up your physical activity in shorter segments of 10 minutes or more.

◆ **Set rewards.** Whether your goal was to be active for 15 minutes a day, to walk farther than you did last week, or simply to stay positive, you deserve recognition for your efforts. Some ideas for rewards include a new CD to motivate you, new walking shoes, or a new outfit.

◆ **Get support.** Get a family member or friend to be physically active with you. It may be more fun, and your buddy can cheer you on and help you stick with it.

◆ **Track progress.** Keep a journal of your physical activity. You may not feel like you are making progress but when you look back at where you started, you may be pleasantly surprised! You can make copies of the blank journal at the end of this booklet to keep track of your efforts.

SAMPLE JOURNAL

Date	Activity	Total Time	Goal	How I Felt
Monday, March 1	Walking Gardening	5 minutes 20 minutes	5 minutes 20 minutes	Difficult, but felt good to finish
Tuesday, March 2	Rest Day			Glad to have a break
Wednesday, March 3	Walking	5 minutes, 2x each	5 minutes	Went with Anne at work—fun!
Thursday, March 4	Walking Stretching	8 minutes 15 minutes	8 minutes 15 minutes	A little difficult to increase...
Friday, March 5	Rest Day			Ready to get active
Saturday, March 6	Walking Stretching	8 minutes 10 minutes	8 minutes 10 minutes	Good way to start the weekend
Sunday, March 7	Chair Dancing Marching in Place	15 minutes 8 minutes	Have fun! 8 minutes	Pumped up the music and got moving!

◆ **Have fun!** Try different activities to find the ones you really enjoy.

What physical activities can a very large person do?

MOST very large people can do some or all of the physical activities in this booklet. You do not need special skills or a lot of equipment. You can do:

◆ **Weight-bearing activities,** like walking and climbing stairs, which involve lifting or pushing your own body weight.

◆ **Nonweight-bearing activities,** like swimming and water workouts, which put less stress on your joints because you do not have to lift or push your own weight. If your feet or joints hurt when you stand, nonweight-bearing activities may be best for you.

◆ **Lifestyle activities,** like gardening or washing the car, which are great ways to get moving. Lifestyle activities do not have to be planned out ahead of time.

Remember that physical activity does not have to be hard or boring to be good for you. Anything that gets you moving around—even for only a few minutes a day—is a healthy start to getting more fit.

Walking (Weight Bearing)

Walking may help you:

◆ Improve your fitness.

◆ Increase the number of calories your body uses.

◆ Increase your energy levels.

Tips for Walking

◆ **Try to walk 5 minutes a day for the first week.** Walk 8 minutes the next week. Stay at 8-minute walks until you feel comfortable. Then increase your walks to 11 minutes. Slowly lengthen each walk, or try walking faster.

◆ **Gradually increase your walks** to give your heart and lungs— as well as your leg muscles—a good workout.

◆ **Wear comfortable walking shoes** with a lot of support. If you walk frequently, you may need to buy new shoes often. You may wish to speak with a podiatrist about when you need to purchase new walking shoes.

◆ **Wear garments that prevent inner-thigh chafing,** such as tights or spandex shorts.

◆ **Make walking fun.** Walk with a friend or pet. Walk in places you enjoy, like a park or shopping mall.

To learn more, read the brochure *Walking...A Step in the Right Direction* from the Weight-control Information Network (WIN). (This publication is available in English and Spanish.)

Do I need to see my health care provider before I start being physically active?

You should talk to your health care provider if you:

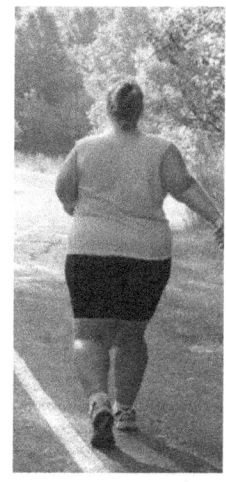

• Have a chronic disease or have risk factors for a chronic disease, such as asthma or diabetes.

- Have high blood pressure, high cholesterol, or a personal or family history of heart disease.
- Are pregnant.
- Are a smoker.
- Are unsure of your health status or have any concerns that exercise might be unsafe for you.

Chances are your health care provider will be pleased with your decision to start an activity program. It is unlikely that you will need a complete medical exam before you go out for a short walk.

Dancing (Weight Bearing or Nonweight Bearing)

Dancing may help:

- Tone your muscles.
- Improve your flexibility.
- Make your heart stronger.
- Make your lungs work better.

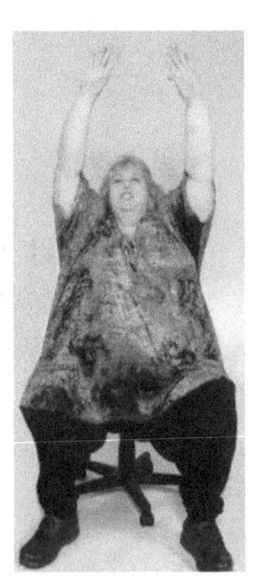

You can dance in a health club, in a nightclub, or at home. To dance at home, just move your body to some lively music!

Dancing on your feet is a weight-bearing activity. Dancing while seated is a nonweight-bearing activity. Sometimes called chair dancing, this activity lets you move your arms and legs to music while taking the weight off your feet. This may be a good choice if you cannot stand on your feet for a long time.

See the list of additional resources at the end of this booklet for seated workout videos.

Water Workouts (Nonweight Bearing)

Exercising in water:

- **Helps flexibility.** You can bend and move your body in water in ways you cannot on land.

- **Reduces risk of injury.** Water makes your body float. This keeps your joints from being pounded or jarred and helps prevent sore muscles and injury.

- **Keeps you refreshed.** You can keep cool in water—even when you are working hard.

You do not need to know how to swim to work out in water—you can do shallow-water or deep-water exercises without swimming.

For **shallow-water workouts,** the water level should be between your waist and your chest. If the water is too shallow, it will be hard to move your arms underwater. If the water is deeper than chest-height, it will be hard to keep your feet on the pool bottom.

For **deep-water workouts,** most of your body is underwater. This means that your whole body will get a good workout. For safety and comfort, wear a foam belt or life jacket.

Many swim centers offer classes in water workouts. Check with the pools in your area to find the best water workout for you.

Where to Work Out

You can do many activities in your home. But there are other fun places to be active, including health clubs, recreation centers, or outdoors. It may be hard to be physically active around other people. Keep in mind that you have just as much right to be healthy and active as anyone else.

Weight Training
(Weight Bearing or Nonweight Bearing)

Weight training may help you:

◆ Build strong muscles and bones. You can weight train at home or at a fitness center.

◆ Increase the number of calories your body uses.

You do not need benches or bars to begin weight training at home. You can use a pair of hand weights or even two soup cans.

To make sure you are using the correct posture, and that your movements are slow and controlled, you may want to schedule a session with a personal trainer. Ask your health care provider for a referral to a personal trainer. You may need to check with your health insurer about whether this service is covered by your plan.

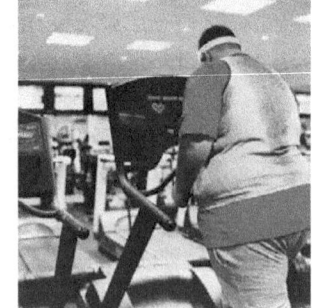

Weight Training Rule of Thumb

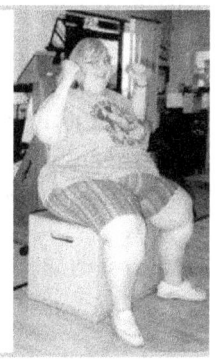

If you cannot lift a weight six times in a row, the weight you are lifting is too heavy. If you can easily lift a weight 15 times in a row, your weight is too light.

If you decide to buy a home gym, check its weight rating (the number of pounds it can support) to make sure it is safe for your size. If you want to join a fitness center where you can use weights, shop around for one where you feel at ease.

See the list of additional resources at the end of this booklet for fitness-related publications.

Bicycling (Nonweight Bearing)

You can bicycle indoors on a stationary bike, or outdoors on a road bike. Biking does not stress any one part of the body—your weight is spread among your arms, back, and hips.

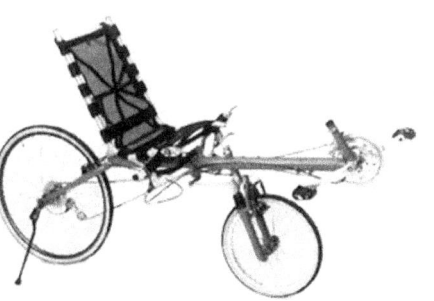

You may want to use a recumbent bike. On this type of bike, you sit low to the ground with your legs reaching forward to the pedals.

Photograph courtesy of Bicycles by Haluzak, Santa Rosa, California

This may feel better than sitting upright. The seat on a recumbent bike is also wider than the seat on an upright bike.

For biking outdoors, you may want to try a mountain bike. These bikes have wider tires and are heavy. You can also buy a larger seat to put on your bike.

Make sure the bike you buy has a weight rating at least as high as your own weight.

Yoga (Weight Bearing or Nonweight Bearing)

Yoga may help you:

◆ Be more flexible.

◆ Feel more relaxed.

◆ Improve posture.

Yoga may help you breathe deeply, relax, and get rid of stress.

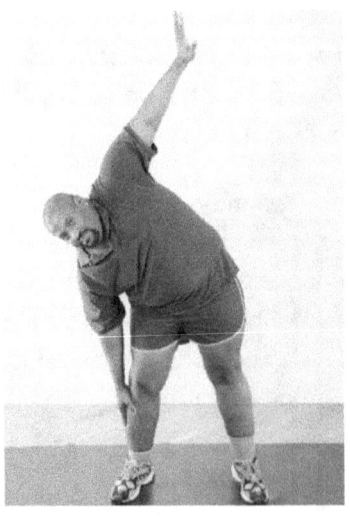

Your local fitness center may offer yoga, tai chi, or other mind/body classes. You may want to start with "gentle" classes, like those aimed at seniors.

See the list of additional resources at the end of this booklet for information about videos and publications for large people.

Questions to Ask When Choosing a Fitness Center

- Can the treadmills or benches support people who are large?
- Does the fitness staff know how to work with people of larger sizes?
- Can I take time to see how I like the center before I sign up?
- Is the aim of signing up to have fun and get healthy?
- What are the center's hours? What time of day is it crowded?

Lifestyle Activities

Lifestyle physical activities do not have to be planned. You can make small changes to make your day more physically active and improve your health. For example:

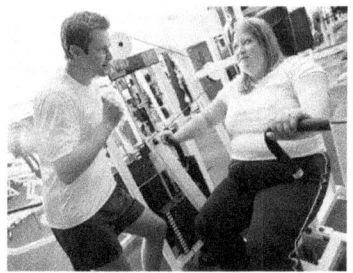

- If possible, take 2- to 3-minute walking breaks at work a few times a day.
- Put away the TV remote control— get up to change the channel.
- March in place during TV commercials.
- Stand or walk, rather than sit, while talking on the phone.
- Play with your family.

Even a shopping trip can be exercise, since it is a chance to walk and carry your bags. In addition, doing chores like lawn mowing, raking leaves, gardening, and housework can count as activity.

Applaud yourself!

If you can do only a few or none of these activities, it is OK. **Appreciate what you can do**, even if you think it is a small amount. Doing any movement—even for a short time—can make you healthier. Remember, each activity you do is a step toward a more active lifestyle.

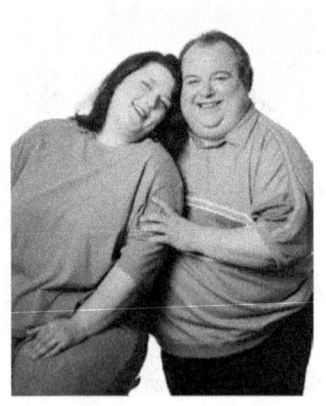

Safety Tips

Tips for Safe Physical Activity

Stop your activity right away if you:

◆ Have pain, tightness, or pressure in your chest or neck, shoulder, or arm.

◆ Feel dizzy or sick.

◆ Break out in a cold sweat.

◆ Have muscle cramps.

◆ Are extremely short of breath.

◆ Feel pain in your joints, feet, ankles, or legs. You could hurt yourself if you ignore the pain.

Ask your health care provider what to do if you have any of these symptoms.

Slow down if you feel out of breath.

The "Talk Test" is an easy way to monitor your physical activity intensity:

◆ You should be able to talk during your activity, without gasping for breath.

◆ When talking becomes difficult, your activity may be too hard.

◆ If talking becomes difficult for you while exercising, slow down until you are able to talk comfortably again.

Wear Suitable Clothes

◆ Wear lightweight, loose-fitting tops so you can move easily.

◆ Wear clothes made of fabrics that absorb sweat and remove it from your skin.

◆ Never wear rubber or plastic suits. Plastic suits could hold the sweat on your skin and make your body overheat.

◆ Women should wear a good support bra.

◆ Wear supportive athletic shoes for weight-bearing activities.

◆ Wear a knit hat to keep you warm when you are physically active outdoors in cold weather. Wear a tightly woven, wide-brimmed hat in hot weather to help keep you cool and protect you from the sun.

◆ Wear sunscreen when you are physically active outdoors.

◆ Wear garments that prevent inner-thigh chafing, such as tights or spandex shorts.

Drink fluids when you are thirsty.

Drink fluids regularly while you are being physically active. Water or other fluids will help keep you hydrated when you are sweating.

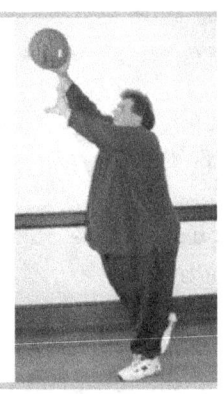

Healthy, fit bodies come in all sizes. Whatever your size or shape, get physically active now and keep moving for a healthier you!

Additional Resources

Note: Inclusion of non-Federal resources is for information only and does not imply endorsement by the Government.

Weight-control Information Network Publications

Changing Your Habits: Steps to Better Health

This fact sheet explains the stages of change and how to work through each stage one step at a time. It focuses on overcoming common barriers to making healthy changes and setting goals to eat healthier and be more physically active. Available from WIN, *http://www.win.niddk.nih.gov/publications/changing-habits.htm*. NIH Publication No. 08–6444. 2008.

Tips to Help You Get Active

This booklet provides ideas and tips for becoming physically active. It focuses on overcoming common barriers and setting goals. Available from WIN, *http://www.win.niddk.nih.gov/publications/tips.htm*. NIH Publication No. 06–5578. 2009.

Walking...A Step in the Right Direction

This pamphlet explains how to start a walking program, presents a sample program, and shows stretches for warming up and cooling down. Available in English and Spanish from WIN, *http://www.win.niddk.nih.gov/publications/walking.htm*. NIH Publication No. 07–4155. 2007.

Fitness-related Publications

Active Living Every Day: 20 Weeks to Lifelong Vitality

Steven N. Blair, Andrea L. Dunn, Bess H. Marcus, Ruth Ann Carpenter, and Peter Jaret. Human Kinetics, 2001. This book offers a step-by-step plan for getting and staying active. The information, suggested activities, and self-help tools in each chapter were successfully tested with people who followed the plan and learned to make activity a part of their daily lives. The 20 chapters correspond to the 20 weeks of the program, but readers are encouraged to go at their own pace. Available from *http:// www.humankinetics.com* or your local or online bookstore.

Great Shape: The First Fitness Guide for Large Women

Pat Lyons and Debby Burgard. iUniverse, 2000. This book urges women to be physically active for fun, fitness, and positive body image instead of for weight loss. The authors describe a healthy lifestyle program including walking, swimming, dancing, martial arts, bicycling, and more. Available from *http://www.iuniverse.com* or your local or online bookstore.

Real Fitness for Real Women: A Unique Workout Program for the Plus-Size Woman

Rochelle Rice. Warner Books, 2001. This book describes a 6-week introductory fitness program that includes warm-ups, aerobics, strength training and stretching techniques, and meditation. Photos of plus-size women demonstrate the exercises. The book also addresses getting motivated, creating support, evaluating current abilities, and increasing self-acceptance. Available from *http://www.rochellerice.com* or your local or online bookstore.

Other Publications and Resources

Plus Size Yellow Pages

Over 3,000 online resources for fitness clothes up to 6X, casual wear up to 10X, bikes, bike seats, kayaks, sports bras, supportive tights/leggings, supportive fitness shoes, and much more.
http://www.plussizeyellowpages.com.

Videos

BIG MOVES: Yoga for Chair and Bed

Mara Nesbitt. This video is designed for people who have difficulty getting down to or up from the floor. Led by a plus-size instructor, it includes stretches done standing, sitting, and lying on a bed, plus a guided meditation. Available from Mirage Video Productions, P.O. Box 19141, Portland, OR 97280; or *http://www.miragevideos.com.*

Chair Dancing

Jodi Stolove. This no-impact video series is designed to improve muscle tone, flexibility, and cardiovascular endurance without putting stress on your knees, back, hips, or feet. Available from Chair Dancing International, Inc., 2658 Del Mar Heights Road, Del Mar, CA 92014; 1–800–551–4386; or *http://www.chairdancing.com*.

Yoga for Round Bodies, Volumes 1 and 2

Linda DeMarco and Genia Pauli Haddon. These videos offer a fitness system based on Kripalu yoga to promote strength, flexibility, stress relief, and cardiovascular health. Round-bodied instructors tailor classic yoga postures to large people at both beginner and intermediate levels in each video. Available from Plus Publications, P.O. Box 265–W, Scotland, CT 06264; 1–800–436–9642; or online retailers.

Organizations and Programs

YMCA and YWCA

The YMCA and YWCA offer physical fitness and health awareness programs in many locations throughout the United States. Contact YMCA of the U.S.A., 101 North Wacker Drive, Chicago, IL 60606; 1–800–872–9622; or *http://www.ymca.net*. Contact YWCA of the U.S.A., 1015 18th Street, NW, Suite 1100, Washington, DC 20036; (202) 467–0801; or *http://www.ywca.org*.

Council on Size and Weight Discrimination, Inc.

The Council on Size and Weight Discrimination, Inc. (CSWD) is a nonprofit organization that seeks to improve heal h care and access to services for large people through educational programs, media monitoring, and medical conference attendance. Contact CSWD at P.O. Box 305, Mount Marion, NY 12456; (845) 679-1209; *http://www.cswd.org*.

National Association to Advance Fat Acceptance

The National Association to Advance Fat Acceptance (NAAFA) is a nonprofit organization that seeks to end discrimination based on body size and to improve the quality of life for large people. It offers a variety of publications and videos on size acceptance, self-esteem, and health and fitness. Contact NAAFA at: P.O. Box 22510, Oakland, CA 94609; (916) 558–6880; or *http://www.naafa.org*.

Websites

U.S. Department of Health and Human Services

Physical Activity Guidelines for Americans. October 2008. Available at *http://www.health.gov/PAGuidelines*.

U.S. Department of Agriculture

ChooseMyPlate. More information and interactive tools on healthy eating and physical activity are available at *http://www.choosemyplate.gov*.

Body Positive®

This site addresses issues ranging from self-esteem to fitness to finding respectful health care providers. It includes resources and links to related sites. *http://www.bodypositive.com*.

Healthy Living with Bliss™

This site includes information on walking, swimming, aerobics, stretching, and other fitness activities for large and very large people. A resource section includes fitness wear, books, exercise equipment, classes, and information on where to buy fitness videos for large people. There is an online workbook, e-newsletter, and a chat with plus-size personal fitness trainer Kelly Bliss. *http://www.kellybliss.com*.

MyStart! Online

MyStart! Online is a personalized, Internet-based program of the American Heart Association designed to help individuals and companies make positive lifestyle changes through walking and eating better. It features free online tools to help you track your daily dietary intake and physical activity, monitor your progress, create personal walking maps, and access health information links and resources. This website also includes a section specifically for companies on how to form a "Start! Worksite Wellness Walking Program." *http://startwalkingnow.org/mystart_tracker.jsp*.

Mayo Clinic Fitness Center

This website contains many different articles about fitness. It offers a set of articles that are all about walking for fitness and includes a shoe-buying guide and a pedometer guide. It also contains slide shows for strength training and stretching exercises. *http://www.mayoclinic.com/health/fitness/SM99999.*

Activity Pledge

Pledging to be active may help you achieve your physical activity goals.

Download and print this pledge from the web and hang it on your refrigerator, calendar, or bulletin board. Using the pledge can help you stay motivated and focus on your activity goals for the week. Also, feel free to download and photocopy the pledge and use it to continue to make activity goals for weeks 5 through 8 and beyond.

My Pledge to Be Active

I, _____, will be physically active for me, so that I may live longer and feel better!

I will work through my barriers to being active!

I will set activity goals and rewards, get support, and track my progress!

I will build up to being more active, and I will choose activities I like to do!

Use the goal-setting card on the following page to help you set weekly activity goals.

My Weekly Activity Goals

Week 1 Goals

I commit to begin _____ (type of
activity) for _____ minutes on:

❑ Monday   ❑ Tuesday   ❑ Wednesday
❑ Thursday   ❑ Friday   ❑ Saturday   ❑ Sunday

Week 2 Goals

I commit to begin _____ (type of
activity) for _____ minutes on:

❑ Monday   ❑ Tuesday   ❑ Wednesday
❑ Thursday   ❑ Friday   ❑ Saturday   ❑ Sunday

Week 3 Goals

I commit to begin _____ (type of
activity) for _____ minutes on:

❑ Monday   ❑ Tuesday   ❑ Wednesday
❑ Thursday   ❑ Friday   ❑ Saturday   ❑ Sunday

Week 4 and Beyond

I commit to begin _____ (type of
activity) for _____ minutes on:

❑ Monday   ❑ Tuesday   ❑ Wednesday
❑ Thursday   ❑ Friday   ❑ Saturday   ❑ Sunday

Sample Activity Journal

Keeping an activity journal is a useful tool to help you stay motivated, stay on track, and reach your goals. It may be helpful to set a short-term goal, a long-term goal, and rewards for meeting those goals.

JOURNAL

Date	Activity	Total Time
Monday		
Tuesday		
Wednesday		
Thursday		
Friday		
Saturday		
Sunday		

You can photocopy this journal page to keep track of your efforts and improvements.

Short-term goal(s):
Long-term goal(s):
Reward(s):

Weight-control Information Network

1 WIN Way
Bethesda, MD 20892–3665
Phone: (202) 828–1025
Toll-free number: 1–877–946–4627
FAX: (202) 828–1028
Email: win@info.niddk.nih.gov
Internet: *http://www.win.niddk.nih.gov*

The Weight-control Information Network (WIN) is a national information service of the National Institute of Diabetes and Digestive and Kidney Diseases (NIDDK) of the National Institutes of Health, which is the Federal Government's lead agency responsible for biomedical research on nutrition and obesity. Authorized by Congress (Public Law 103–43), WIN provides the general public, health professionals, the media, and Congress with up-to-date, science-based health information on weight control, obesity, physical activity, and related nutritional issues.

Publications produced by WIN are reviewed by both NIDDK scientists and outside experts. This publication was also reviewed by:

Steven Blair, P.E.D., Department of Exercise Science, Arnold School of Public Health, University of South Carolina.

John M. Jakicic, Ph.D., Chair, Department of Health and Physical Activity, Director, Physical Activity and Weight Management Research Center, University of Pittsburgh.

Special thanks to the Women of Substance Health Spa, Kelly Bliss, M.Ed., and Rochelle Rice, M.A., of In Fitness and In Health for providing many of the photographs in this brochure.

NIH Publication No. 10–4352
Updated February 2010